Mauricio Ferreira e Silva Farco

Natural Feeding for an Adult Dog

Mauricio Ferreira e Silva Farco

Natural Feeding for an Adult Dog

Nutritional Aspects of a Natural Diet

ScienciaScripts

Imprint

Any brand names and product names mentioned in this book are subject to trademark, brand or patent protection and are trademarks or registered trademarks of their respective holders. The use of brand names, product names, common names, trade names, product descriptions etc. even without a particular marking in this work is in no way to be construed to mean that such names may be regarded as unrestricted in respect of trademark and brand protection legislation and could thus be used by anyone.

Cover image: www.ingimage.com

This book is a translation from the original published under ISBN 978-613-9-67088-8.

Publisher:
Sciencia Scripts
is a trademark of
Dodo Books Indian Ocean Ltd. and OmniScriptum S.R.L publishing group

120 High Road, East Finchley, London, N2 9ED, United Kingdom
Str. Armeneasca 28/1, office 1, Chisinau MD-2012, Republic of Moldova, Europe
Printed at: see last page
ISBN: 978-620-8-10845-8

Copyright © Mauricio Ferreira e Silva Farco
Copyright © 2024 Dodo Books Indian Ocean Ltd. and OmniScriptum S.R.L publishing group

SUMMARY

ACKNOWLEDGMENTS

First of all, I would like to thank God, who allows us to exist on this Earth. To my parents who have always been by my side, supported me in my choices and made it possible for me to study in the city of Porto Alegre. To this institution, UFRGS, which made my training as a Veterinary Doctor possible. And to the professors and professionals, for all their wise teachings, especially Professor Ana Cristina Pacheco de Araujo and professional Wanessa Beheregaray, who guided me in the construction of this course conclusion.

SUMMARY

Because they are carnivorous and opportunistic animals, they became close to hunters and over the years developed a closer relationship with humans. Nowadays, dogs are completely dependent on people, limited to domestic homes, and feed on what humans offer them. For practical reasons, more and more owners are feeding their animals commercial, processed food.

This course conclusion aims to analyze the behavioral and nutritional aspects of dogs and describe a complete homemade diet for an adult dog. It offers the possibility of feeding dogs in a more natural but safe way. With fresh ingredients, closer to what they would eat in the wild, without the addition of industrial chemicals and preservatives. Natural feeding brings many benefits, both physiological and behavioral, as long as the owner is willing to dedicate a little more time to their dog.

Keywords: dogs, nutrition, ingredients, feeding;

1 - INTRODUCTION

Food (nutrition) is of paramount importance for the maintenance of life, the formation of tissues, metabolic processes, enzymatic reactions and the immune system. It is necessary for the maintenance of a healthy physiological state, and serves as a support for recovery from pathological states. The effects that food can have on dogs are diverse, ranging from blood parameters that are affected by the metabolism of proteins (levels of urea and plasma creatinine), lipids and carbohydrates to factors linked to urinary pH (formation of uroliths), fecal quality, microbiological parameters, the animal's general appearance and behavior (MEEKER, 2006).

Compared to (commercial) feed, dry extruded feed and pasty (wet) feed, natural feed, properly balanced, offers nutrients with higher digestibility rates, greater acceptability by the animals, improves the general appearance of the feces, reduces water consumption, among other benefits, in addition to not containing artificial substances such as preservatives, dyes and flavorings. (FRANÇA, 2009)

However, it is important to know the needs of each nutrient correctly, so that it is possible to prepare a "balanced" diet, with a margin of safety in the proportion of ingredients, in order to avoid any nutritional deficiencies. Animal products such as meat, eggs and even meaty bones, as well as human foods such as grains, cereals, legumes, vegetables and even fruit, are normally used in natural diets. In addition to supplementation, which can be done through natural products such as oils of plant and animal origin and dairy products.

All the stages involved in preparing the diet are important, from the choice of ingredients, which must be quality products and in good condition, through processing, cooking and handling, and storage, by refrigerating or freezing. This type of food definitely requires the owner to have more time available for preparing the diet, as well as attention to the choice of ingredients and the care needed to reduce the risk of microbiological contamination.

The aim of this final project is to clarify the benefits and define a natural diet for an adult dog, i.e. with selected ingredients, minimal processing and no artificial additives, taking into account nutritional needs, specific physiological and pathological conditions and some of the particularities of dogs with regard to diet.

2 - CANES, CHARACTERISTICS OF THE SPECIES

The relationship between man and dog began approximately 15,000 years ago. When man fed the canines during hunting seasons in exchange for protection from the camps at night. Man selected these wild canines for favorable characteristics, such as submissive behavior, keen senses to accompany the hunt and an instinct for protection. Thus began the process of selecting and domesticating dogs. Fifteen thousand years of racial selection may have changed some of the superficial characteristics and behavior of dogs, but inside them, virtually nothing has changed. Dry food diets, rich in carbohydrates, have been created in the last 80 - 100 years. On the evolutionary scale, this doesn't seem like a significant amount of time compared to the thousands of years that dogs have demonstrated their carnivorous nature. In 1993, the Smithsonian Natural History Museum and the American Society of Mammalogists, after DNA tests comparing *Canis lupus* (wolf) with *Canis familiaris* (dog), renamed the dog, *Canis lupus familiaris*, as a subspecies of the wolf. The results showed that the domestic dog arose from 26 gray wolf populations, and that the dog is twenty times more closely related to the wolf than coyotes (*Canis latrans*). The dog, a highly evolved predator, is included in the order Carnivora (GODFREY & RUISH, 2001).

2.1 - Anatomical and physiological aspects

Almost 15,000 years of domestication have not been enough to turn dogs (*Canis familiaris*) into complete omnivores, they retain the characteristics that classify them as carnivores, with some authors classifying them as semi-carnivores. They have jaws designed for cutting, with a dentition made up of 42 teeth and very short chewing; few taste buds, dogs don't have a very sharp palate; little or no pre-digestion by saliva; a stomach adapted to swallowing prey quickly, it can hold large volumes, with an acidic stomach pH (1 to 2) that destroys pathogenic microorganisms; with a relatively short digestive tract, the length of the small intestine varies from 2 to 6 m depending on the size of the dog, the transit time is only about 2 hours, the transit in the large intestine is very slow, even though it is short (20 to 80 cm), it is in this organ that the fermentation of undigested food takes place. Fundamentally active animals derive the energy they need from fats and proteins. They don't have the "cholesterol" problems that humans do, but they can suffer from obesity if their diet is not respected (GRANDJEAN, 2006).

2.2 - Eating Behavior

Domestic dogs usually eat a lot when presented with a very palatable food for the first time, or in large quantities. But when restricted to dry diets, they may eat very little several times, with 10 to 13 meals, most of them during the day. Their behavior pattern is no different from that of wolves, who are excellent hunters and take down large prey, even larger than themselves. Being able to go for long periods without feeding, when a fresh carcass is available they eat large quantities in one go. Most of the time, however, wolves rely on small, frequent meals throughout the day, eating small mammals, reptiles, insects, fruit and other varieties of plant matter (WILLS & SIMPSON, 1994).

Most animals, including dogs, fed *ad libitum*, regulate the amount of food until they reach a set weight, i.e. according to the amount of energy consumed. After a period of deprivation, animals overeat until their weight is adjusted. Dogs with access to highly palatable food set a higher consumption limit, but this varies according to the individual and the breed. *Beagles*, for example, gain more weight with more palatable diets than *Terriers* (WILLS & SIMPSON, 1994).

2.3 - Aberrant behavior

Cats and dogs eat grass and other types of plants. Why they do this is unclear. Grass and other plants are not readily digested and may irritate the gastrointestinal tract, resulting in vomiting. However, some domestic animals consume grass without vomiting, and perhaps only ingest this plant matter for its taste and texture (SCHENCK, 2010).

Dogs have a tendency to "go through the garbage". This behavior is probably normal; dogs like the taste of certain substances produced by rotting food. Unfortunately, rotting food can contain high amounts of bacteria, which, if ingested, can be pathogenic. Ingesting garbage can result in vomiting, diarrhea, abdominal pain, shock and even death. Access to garbage should be avoided (SCHENCK, 2010).

Coprophagia is the ingestion of feces by dogs. Sometimes dogs ingest their own feces, but more often they ingest the feces of other animals, including other species. This condition is much more common in dogs than in cats. Coprophagy is a normal behavior in females, who ingest the feces of their puppies in the first three weeks of life, in order to leave the area clean and to distract attention from predators. In the wild, canines also have a habit of ingesting the feces of herbivores, perhaps because it is rich in certain nutrients. Potential causes of coprophagia include intestinal parasites, intestinal malabsorption, hyperthyroidism, Cushing's disease, diabetes mellitus or steroid administration. Complications associated with coprophagia include gastroenteritis and diarrhea, especially if bovine feces are consumed, as well as reinfection with intestinal parasites. The best treatment for coprophagia is to prevent exposure to feces (SCHENCK, 2010).

3 - FEEDING THE DOGS

The effects that food can have on dogs are diverse, ranging from blood parameters, which are affected by the metabolism of proteins (levels of urea and plasma creatinine), lipids and carbohydrates, to factors linked to urinary pH (formation of uroliths), fecal quality, microbiological parameters, the general appearance of the animal and behavior (MEEKER, 2006).

According to Borges & Saad (2004), when formulating diets for dogs and cats, whether homemade or commercial, some key points must be respected so that the end product is of high quality: formulation appropriate to the nutritional needs of each physiological phase of the animal (percentage composition); quantitative balance between nutrients; correct ratio between lipids, proteins, carbohydrates, minerals and vitamins; the origin of the ingredients; the use of functional foods that increase the dietary value; palatability and the appropriate preparation process.

Inappropriate nutrition can result in the development of a wide variety of nutritional imbalances in dogs, which can even lead to clinical illness. However, nutritional deficiencies are most commonly observed in growing animals. Adult animals in a state of maintenance are less prone to nutritional deficiencies, due to their body reserves and comparatively low requirements. The development of nutritional diseases in adult animals takes several weeks or even months to be observed, however, they can have serious consequences (WILLS & SIMPSON, 2006).

In a study comparing the adequacy of homemade and commercial diets, calcium, the Ca:P ratio, and vitamins A and E are below the recommendations in most homemade diets. So are the concentrations of potassium, copper and zinc. Feeding unbalanced diets can lead to complications such as osteodystrophy, osteopenia and secondary nutritional hyperparathyroidism. Meat products, which are usually the basis of homemade diets, have high phosphorus concentrations and low calcium levels. If no source of calcium is added to the diet, with an inadequate supply of calcium, the Ca:P ratio becomes very low. Secondary nutritional hyperparathyroidism occurs when there is a high concentration of parathyroid hormone, increasing serum calcium levels and resulting in a decrease in bone density. Vitamin D deficiency can lead to rickets, characterized by osteodystrophy. Calcium and vitamin D deficiencies are especially problematic in puppies and growing dogs, which require an adequate balance of calcium and phosphorus for bone growth. Some ingredients can be very rich in certain nutrients, such as vitamins, and cause problems if they are not properly balanced. Diets based on liver can lead to vitamin A poisoning. Some recipes may contain ingredients that are offered raw; these ingredients may contain bacteria that would be destroyed by cooking. The practice of feeding raw ingredients is discouraged by some authors (SCHENCK, 2010).

According to some studies, the ingredients used to make animal feed vary in their ability to provide the animal with nutrients. The digestible content of nutrients in the final feed is important to ensure that an animal can absorb enough nutrients from the diet to meet its needs (HENDRIKSAN & SRITHEREN, 2002). Therefore, a balanced feed must contain highly digestible ingredients, resulting in a greater supply of nutrients to meet the nutritional demands of the animal's tissues.

In the same way that digestibility affects the availability of nutrients, it also alters the volume and shape of feces. As the digestibility of the diet increases, fecal volume decreases considerably. A highly digestible food produces solid, well-formed feces (CASE et al., 1998).

3.1 - Natural Food

The term "natural" covers food without chemicals or artificial preservatives. According to The European Pet Food Industry Federation, FEDIAF, a stricter definition would be: pet food components without any additives and which have only undergone processing to make them suitable for pet food production and maintain the content of all essential nutrients. Examples of processing include: freezing, concentration, cooking and pasteurization (GROOT & SCHEREUDER, 2009).

According to Groot & Schreuder (2009), the number of pet food manufacturers starting out in this market and the profile of pet owners who associate themselves with these types of products on a strategic level are increasing rapidly. According to consumers, environmental and health benefits are the main factors for purchasing this type of product.

According to Freeman & Michel (2001), diets or raw foods can be separated into three basic categories: (1) complete (balanced) raw food diets, typically sold frozen; they claim to be complete and balanced, subject to regulation by the *American Association of Feed Control Officials* (AAFCO); (2) homemade complete raw food diets, which require the owner to prepare the recipe (available in books and articles, as well as on the internet); the ingredients of these homemade diets can be completely varied, depending on the person who formulated the recipe; many of them are balanced overall; however, each individual meal may not be balanced and (3) combination diets consisting of commercially available grain and supplement mixtures offered in combination with the raw meat provided by the owner. These diets are not subject to regulation.

3.1.1- Advantages and disadvantages

Feeding dogs natural ingredients has advantages and disadvantages. Some positive points are: the offer of natural food, without the addition of artificial substances such as colorings, flavorings and preservatives; greater availability of nutrients, due to the higher quality of the ingredients; improvement in fecal score, related to the quality of proteins and starch content; and maintenance of urinary pH, in a range to prevent uroliths; (FRANÇA, 2009). They also offer additional advantages such as greater acceptability for dogs (greater palatability), and the possibility of using functional foods which, as well as nourishing, act in a preventative manner and even in the treatment of illnesses.

According to França (2009), for crude protein and ethereal extract, treatments with natural foods show a similar or higher nutritional value than commercial foods classified as super-premium,   possibly due to the use of by-products, unlike natural foods made up of ingredients intended for human consumption, which have a higher biological value. Among the disadvantages of this type of feeding, we can mention, in addition to the risks of a poorly formulated diet, the greater time dedicated to feeding the animal by the owner, i.e. the time needed to choose and buy the ingredients, as well as the stages of food processing, such as cooking (if any), fractioning and storage.

In addition to the nutritional value, the quality or food safety of the final product is of paramount importance, since all risks of contamination with the products and raw materials must be avoided during production (GROOT & SCHEREUDER, 2009).

As with conventional pet food, the use of raw natural food for dogs and cats does not exempt the owner from food safety risks. The risks of biological contamination, especially salmonellosis, toxoplasmosis and various worms, are the weak points of natural raw diets. The possibilities for reducing and controlling the biological contamination to which raw natural foods are subject include measures involving processing, such as pasteurization, cooking, radiation and dehydration (SAAD & JOSÉ, 2008).

3.2 - Commercial food

Dogs have an omnivorous eating habit compared to cats, which allows them greater scope in the selection of ingredients for formulation, as well as the ability to adapt to commercial feeds, which differ greatly in their composition, ingredients, texture and form (NRC, 2006).

Commercial foods vary in their formulation and processing, with different ingredients, which can vary in composition and, consequently, affect their use by animals, as well as causing different physiological and metabolic responses in the animal organism. They are formulated with cereal grains, products derived from cereal grains, products derived from soya beans, animal by-products, products derived from animal sources (including milk derivatives), fats and oils, vitamins and micro- and macro-minerals. Commercially, dry food for dogs and cats can be classified as economy, standard, premium and superpremium (CASE et al., 1998).

On the other hand, natural foods can be made up of ingredients intended for human consumption, seeking to approximate the composition of foods that animals obtain in the wild, with a greater contribution of ingredients such as protein and lipids to these animals. (FRANÇA, 2009)

Commercial dry feeds require preservatives and antioxidants to prevent oxidative deterioration and the rancidification process. Some natural brands tend to use healthier choices, such as vitamin C (ascorbic acid) and vitamin E, although they provide a much shorter shelf life for the product. In contrast, commercial feeds use synthetic preservatives such as Butylated Hydroxyanisole (BHA) and Butylated Hydroxytoluene (BHT), which can extend shelf life by up to a year. There is concern, however, because some studies have suggested that these substances are carcinogenic. Another synthetic preservative whose long-term safety in dogs has yet to be proven is Ethoxyquinine. Some reports have described altered liver and kidney function in dogs with prolonged use of this substance. Although the Food and Drug Administration (USA) has concluded that the additive does not pose a health threat. In 1997, the US government agency reduced the amount of ethoxyquin allowed in dog food (FLAIM, 2012).

4 - **Nutritional needs**

Table 1 - Minimum requirements for dogs in maintenance (per kilo).

Nutrients	Unit	Quantity
Arginine	mg	21
Histidine	mg	22
Isoleucine	mg	48
Leucine	mg	84
Lysine	mg	50
Methionine - tank	mg	30
Phenylalanine-tyrosine	mg	86
Threonine	mg	44
Tryptophan	mg	13
Valine	mg	60
Crude Fat	g	1
Linoleic acid	mg	200
Càlcio	mg	119
Phosphorus	mg	89
Ca: P ratio	mg	1:1
Potassium	mg	89
Sodium	mg	11
Chlorine	mg	17
Magnesium	mg	8,2
Iron	mg	0,65
Copper	mg	0,06
Manganese	mg	0,1
Zinc	mg	0,72
Iodine	mg	0,0012
Selenium	mg	2,2
Vitamin A	UI	75
Vitamin D	UI	8
Vitamin E	UI	0,5
Thiamine	µg	20
Riboflavin	µg	50
Pantothenic Acid	µg	200
Niacin	µg	225
Pyridoxine	µg	22
Folic acid	µg	4
Vitamin B12	µg	0,5
Hill	mg	25

Source: Adapted from National Research Council (2006).

4.1 - Water

Water is the most important nutrient for dogs, as it is for all living creatures. Dogs obtain water in liquid form from food and from the oxidation of hydrogen during metabolism (metabolic water). Around 10 to 16 g of metabolic water are produced for every 100 kcal of energy metabolized. A dog consuming 2000 kcal of metabolizable energy per day (e.g. German Sheperd) will produce 200 to 320 g of metabolic water. (POND & CHURCH, 2005).

Water is released from the breakdown of food during digestion. The amount of water depends on the type of feed; for example, commercial dry feeds may contain only 6% moisture, commercial wet feeds contain up to 82% moisture. Natural diets, composed of fresh ingredients, generally contain a high moisture content (EDNEY, 1989).

4.2 - Energy

Energy is used to carry out cellular work, processes such as breathing and the activity needed to maintain body temperature. Like humans, dogs maintain a temperature close to 40°C, which requires large amounts of energy. The energy density of the diet must be high enough to provide sufficient calories and maintain an adequate energy balance. It is the main factor that determines the amount of food to be consumed each day (EDNEY, 1989).

Dogs, like other mammals, are not entirely efficient at obtaining energy from food. Therefore, energy intake is studied at three different levels: gross energy (BE), digestible energy (DE) and metabolizable energy (ME). BE is the total amount of energy released in the complete oxidation of the food, determined in a calorimetric pump. Even though a given substance may have a high ME value, it can be unhelpful to dogs if they cannot digest and absorb it. The amount digested and absorbed is called ED and is equal to EB minus the energy released in the feces. Not all the energy absorbed is used by the tissues, as some is lost through the kidneys in the urine. The energy finally used by the tissues is called ME and is calculated by subtracting ED from the energy released in the urine (EDNEY, 1989).

The energy requirements of dogs are commonly expressed in units of metabolisable energy (ME), and small dogs have higher ME requirements per kilo of live weight than large dogs. To explain this difference, the National Research Council (2004) has expressed the requirement of dogs of different sizes per unit of metabolic weight (W= kg to the power of 0.75). The exponent used in the expression is not universally agreed (Case et al, 2000), but the NRC (2004) concludes that an adult dog at maintenance has a ME requirement of 130 kcal/ Wkg 0.75/day. Maintenance requirements may be higher in adolescent or young adult dogs and adult Great Danes and Terriers. They may be lower in dogs that are not very active, elderly dogs or Newfoundland dogs (NRC, 2004). Working, exercising or lactating adult dogs may have a two to three times higher requirement. Dogs of different breeds, temperaments, body condition, or subjected to extreme environments, exercise, or stress, vary on average, the food offered must be subject to individual variations (POND & CHURCH, 2005).

5 - Macronutrients

They are the nutrients present in high quantities in the diet, supplying energy and structural needs. They are proteins, lipids and carbohydrates (EDNEY, 1989).

5.1 - Proteins and amino acids

Proteins are composed of carbon, hydrogen and oxygen, but unlike lipids and fatty acids, they contain nitrogen. Most proteins also contain sulphur. Proteins are large molecules made up of chains of hundreds and even thousands of small subunits called amino acids. Although there are only 22 amino acids in the composition of proteins, the variety of sequences in which they can be arranged is almost infinite, which determines the great variety of proteins that exist in nature. (EDNEY, 1989)

Dogs need protein from their diet to obtain specific amino acids that their tissues cannot synthesize quickly enough. Amino acids are used to form new proteins that are essential for living cells, in which they regulate metabolic processes (in the form of enzymes), form cell structure and are necessary for tissue growth and renewal (EDNEY, 1989).

Therefore, protein requirements vary depending on the dog's age, as well as factors such as stress, growth, pregnancy, lactation and state of health. Healthy adult dogs need approximately 2 g of protein of high biological value per weight (kg)/day. The protein requirement of the diet is satisfied when the dog's metabolic needs for amino acids and nitrogen are met. According to AAFCO, dogs have a requirement of 18% protein in dry matter for maintenance and 22% for growth and reproduction (SCHENCK, 2010).

Without sufficient fat in the diet or energy from carbohydrates, the proteins normally used for growth or maintaining body functions are converted into energy less efficiently. Too little biological protein in the diet, in relation to the energy density, can cause an apparent protein deficiency. Signs produced by protein deficiency or an inappropriate ratio of protein to calories can include: weight loss, skeletal muscle atrophy, dull and brittle hair, anorexia, apathy, reproductive problems, persistent infection, vaccine failure, and failure to respond to treatments. (KAHN, 2010)

A higher protein content in certain diets is based on increased antibody production, greater resistance in the event of physical exertion, rapid replenishment of organic reserves in times of need (pregnancy, lactation and illness), lower feed intake and adequate muscle formation during the growth phase (SEIXAS ET AL, 2003).

With a high protein intake, a possible overload of the organs involved in protein metabolism must be considered, especially the kidneys and liver. Since the amine radical is transformed into ammonia and then into urea, which is then eliminated in the urine by the kidneys (FRANÇA, 2009).

5.1.1-- Essential amino acids

Amino acids, the components of proteins, are classified into two groups: essential and non-essential. Essential amino acids cannot be synthesized by the body in sufficient quantities and must therefore be present in the diet.

According to Pond & Church (2005) the essential amino acids required in puppy and adult dog food are: Methionine and Cystine, Arginine, Histidine, Isoleucine, Leucine, Lysine, Threonine, Phanylalanine, Tryptophan and Valine.

The deficiency of one essential amino acid forces the deamination of the others in proportion to the limitation, preventing the complete synthesis of the necessary proteins. On the other hand, this deamination causes an energy imbalance in the diet, since the tertiary radicals formed in this process will be used to synthesize energy (KAHN, 2010).

5.1.1.1 - Sulfur Amino Acids: Methionine and Cystine

Only methionine is considered an essential amino acid. However, if enough cystine is supplied, methionine can be spared for other functions. The metabolism of sulphur amino acids produces sulphuric acid, which is eliminated in the urine. This is why the natural diet of carnivores rich in sulphur amino acids tends to produce a more acidic urine. Sulphur amino acids are essential for the synthesis of the main protein in the hair, keratin. A lack of sulphur amino acids results in hair loss, delayed growth and a dull, brittle coat. The synthesis required to maintain the skin and coat can account for up to 30% of an adult dog's daily protein requirements.

Generally speaking, sulphur amino acids are present in large quantities in protein sources of animal origin. These aa are therefore rarely lacking in dog diets, with the exception of unsupplemented vegetarian diets. Methionine and cystine are particularly abundant in egg proteins, fish and milk casein. Wheat and corn gluten are also rich in methionine and cystine (GRANDJEAN, 2006).

5.1.1.2 - Arginine

Arginine is an essential amino acid for dogs. Newborn puppies fed on mother's milk lacking in arginine quickly develop cataracts, which is the cause of blindness in some dogs. Arginine is also a precursor of nitric oxide (NO), which plays a relaxing role on the smooth muscle fibers of the vessels.

Arginine has been shown to reduce respiratory problems caused by increased CO2 production during exertion in people suffering from severe chronic heart failure. Arginine also plays a role in immune mechanisms (GRANDJEAN, 2006).

Earlier, Rose and Rice (1939) suggested that adult dogs did not require dietary levels of arginine. However, Burns et al (1981) concluded that adult dogs fed diets "free" of arginine were vomiting due to high blood levels of ammonia as a result of the inability to metabolize nitrogenous compounds (urea cycle) due to the absence of arginine (POND & CHURCH, 2005).

It is abundant in animal tissues such as muscles, skin and fur. Gelatine is very rich in arginine (GRANDJEAN, 2006).

5.1.1.3 - Taurine

Taurine enables the liver to synthesize bile salts. But it also influences the flow of calcium between the inside and outside of the cell, which allows it to act on cardiac function. It also plays an important antioxidant role in the cell. Finally, taurine plays the role of precursor in the synthesis of complex lipids in the skin (glycosphingolipids) which have microbial properties (GRANDJEAN, 2006).

Taurine is believed to be synthesized in the body, in adequate quantities, by the liver of most dogs if sufficient levels of the precursor sulphur amino acids (Methionine and Cystine) are found in the diet (POND & CHURCH, 2005).

Meat is a rich natural source of taurine (GRANDJEAN, 2006).

5.1.1.4 - Lysine

Lysine is an essential amino acid for the dog: it must be supplied by the diet to allow all the proteins in the body to be synthesized. A lysine deficit in a puppy can cause growth retardation, for example.

Lysine is very sensitive to heat: very aggressive heat treatment causes a reaction with sugars (Mailard reaction) which makes lysine unavailable to the body.

It is abundant in animal proteins, especially in meat and milk casein. Soy proteins also contain it in abundance. On the other hand, lysine may be deficient in a diet based on the use of cereals, requiring a supplement of this amino acid (GRANDJEAN, 2006).

5.1.1.5 . - Tyrosine and Phenylalanine

The color of the coat depends on the presence of pheomelanin (yellow to red pigments) and eumelanin (brown to black pigments). The production of these pigments requires the presence of aromatic amino acids (due to their cyclic structure) tyrosine and phenylalanine. A lack of these aa in animals with dark or black coats makes the coat reddish. Studies carried out on dogs of the Newfoundland and black Labrador breeds have shown that the levels of phenylalanine and tyrosine required for optimal pigmentation of the coat are more than 2 times higher than the requirements for growth. Tyrosine supplementation can even increase the color intensity of the coat.

In addition to its role in pigmenting the coat and iris, tyrosine is also a precursor of dopamine, noradrenaline and adrenaline. These molecules are involved in the proper functioning of the brain and reproductive function. Adequate tyrosine supplementation therefore has a positive effect on fertility.

Milk and milk products are excellent sources of tyrosine, as is meat. As for vegetable sources, only rice contains non-negligible amounts of this amino acid (GRANDJEAN, 2006).

5.1.1.6 - Branched-chain amino acids (BCAAs)

Leucine, Isoleucine and Valine

The body is unable to synthesize sufficient quantities of leucine, isoleucone and valine; meeting requirements depends on dietary intake. The blood concentrations of these three amino acids vary according to dietary intake more than the other amino acids. They are able to stimulate the synthesis of proteins and slow down their degradation in the muscles. This property has been attributed specifically to leucine, which is as effective on its own as it is in combination with isoleucine and valine.

AACRs help increase lean mass and prevent muscle atrophy in animals with cancer cachexia. Clinical studies in humans have shown a relationship between AACR supplementation and increased survival time. Valine, leucine and isoleucine represent at least a third of the essential amino acids that make up muscle proteins (GRANDJEAN, 2006).

5.1.1.7 - Protein sources

According to Seixas et al (2003) and Anfal Pet (2008), protein sources for dog food can be classified into two categories: vegetable origin - which includes grains and bran from by-products of industrial processes involving grains and vegetables, and animal origin, which comes from animal tissues or by-products of the chicken, beef, pork, sheep, fish, egg, milk and etc. industries. Protein sources of animal origin are important raw materials in dog diets. However, the variability in their composition and nutritional quality, related to the origin of the raw materials, the ash content and the temperature used in processing, which can reduce the digestibility of the food, must be taken into account (ANFAL PET, 2008).

Table 2. Percentage of nutrients in animal products.

DRY MATERIAL

Products of animal origin	U (%)	MS (%)	EM1 (Kcal)	EM1 (Kcal/g)	PB (%)	MM (%)	EE (%)

Beef	75,0	25,0	130	5,0	70,0	3,5	22,0
Heart bovine	75,6	26,4	135	5,11	68,6	3,2	25,3
Lungs cattle	79,0	21,0	100	4,76	79,1	3,8	16,7
Bovine kidneys	77,7	22,3	113	5,07	75,3	5,4	17,9
Beef liver	73,6	26,4	130	4,92	75,8	4,4	17,1
Chicken (complete)	73,3	26,7	140	5,23	47,4	---	39,8
Eggs in shell	67,0	33,0	142	4,3	33,03	4,5	30,3
Shelled eggs	74,8	25,2	147	5,83	48,8	0	43,3
Fish (sardines)	71 -73	27 -29	119-174	4,4-6,0	46-69	6,2-10	20-46

1 Metabolizable energy (ME) values for humans, (-) Lack of reliable data, U = moisture, ME = metabolizable energy; DM = dry matter; CP = crude protein; MM = mineral matter; EE = ethereal extract. Source: Adapted from França, 2009.

According to Seixas et al (2003), the biological value of protein can be used to assess its quality in pet food. This value corresponds to the fraction absorbed and not excreted by the body, and is related to the digestibility of the protein used in the diet. The biological value of a protein is closely related to

the amount of essential amino acids that this source contains. It is important that the essential amino acids are present in the diet in the correct quantity, as the limitation of one of them will impair the use of the others, since there is a correlation between the proportions and quantities of amino acids for the synthesis of the various proteins that the body will form. Eggs have been given the highest biological value, followed by organ meats, which have a higher biological value than meat from skeletal muscles (FRANÇA, 2009).

According to Bednar et al (200), Seixas et al (2003) and Carciofi (2008), there are variations in the chemical composition of plant protein sources, but they are relatively minor compared to animal sources. However, they contain anti-nutritional factors such as enzyme inhibitors, lectins, tannins, phytates, non-starch polysaccharides, among others, which, when present, can negatively influence the availability of their nutrients.

According to Aldrich (2009), fresh meat would be the preferred material in commercial pet food formulations, but this is not always practiced, for various reasons: expenses associated with freezing and refrigeration; expenses involved with transporting raw materials with a high moisture content; the extrusion process does not support more than 25% fresh meat in the composition of commercial pet food. Therefore, the use of dry feed with concentrated protein is often necessary.

5.2 - Lipids and fatty acids

From a chemical point of view, food fats are basically composed of triglycerides, which are combinations of three fatty acids joined to a glycerol molecule. The differences between fats are due to the different fatty acids that make them up. There are numerous fatty acids in food, characterized in their structure by the number of carbon atoms and double bonds. Saturated fatty acids don't have double bonds and are only a source of energy, while unsaturated fatty acids have one or more double bonds and can therefore be called polyunsaturated and have structural roles (in membranes or blood lipoproteins). Most fats have both types in different proportions (EDNEY, 1988).

Dietary lipids contribute approximately 8.5 kcal ME per gram, about 2.25 times more energy than a gram of carbohydrate. The digestibility of fats is usually high and can be more than 90%. Due to their high energy density, when compared to carbohydrates and proteins, dietary lipids contribute significantly to the energy supply for dogs (FRANÇA, 2009).

As most animals eat to satisfy their caloric needs, a high-fat diet will reduce the amount of food they eat. Lipids are important for meeting the energy needs of very active dogs, workers, sled dogs and lactating dogs. Fat also contributes to the palatability and texture of the diet. As well as providing energy, fat is also important for the absorption of fat-soluble vitamins such as A, D, E and K. Domestic dogs that are not very active or even sedentary do not require high levels of lipids in their diet for maintenance. Very palatable diets rich in fat contribute to increased consumption and obesity. Excess fat in feed can "oppress" digestion and cause steatorrhea (passage of undigested fat), as well as reducing food consumption, which can lead to deficiencies in other nutrients, such as proteins, minerals and vitamins (SCHENCK, 1999).

According to Kahn (2010), low-fat diets are not very palatable, and essential fatty acid deficiency is uncommon in dogs, occurring after long periods of low intake. Adequate diets have adequate fat levels, but when they are stored inappropriately they can result in fatty acid deficiency. Oxidation of fatty acids can occur in foods exposed to high temperatures or in conditions of high humidity. This process is called *rancification*.

In commercial diets, antioxidants are usually added to help prevent lipid oxidation. Homemade diets generally don't have antioxidant additives (preservatives), should be made in small portions and stored properly (KAHN, 2010).

High consumption of fatty acids by dogs is relatively safe. In humans, high consumption can result in atherosclerosis. However, due to the great difference in lipoprotein metabolism, dogs rarely develop atherosclerosis, unless there is already an alteration in lipid metabolism (e.g. hypothyroidism and diabetes mellitus) (KAHN, 2010).

Feeding excess fat can potentially lead to pancreatitis, but this association is unclear. Some dogs with pancreatitis have a history of eating a diet rich in lipids or consuming leftover fatty meat (KAHN, 2010).

Dogs have a minimum requirement for essential fatty acids in their diet. These are polyunsaturated fatty acids, from the Omega 3 and 6 series, which have special functions and cannot be synthesized by the body. In dogs, these are linoleic acid and linolenic acid (SCHENCK, 1999).

Fats from different sources vary greatly in their concentration of omega 3 and 6 fatty acids (EDNEY, 1989).

5.2.1-- Omega 3 fatty acids

The fatty acids of the omega-3 series constitute a particular family in the category of polyunsaturated fatty acids. This family derives from a fatty acid, made up of 18 carbon atoms and 3 double chemical bonds, called alpha-linolenic acid (ALA). Two other longer but very important fatty acids, called Eicosapentaenoic Acid (EPA) and Docosahexaenoic Acid (DHA), are derived from the latter.

The functions of omega-3 fatty acids are numerous, among them: anti-inflammatory role, inhibiting the synthesis of certain chemical mediators of inflammation; improvement in sports performance and cerebral oxygenation (elderly animals); improvements in learning capacity in young animals; (GRANDJEAN, 2006).

Below is a table of different fats and oils with their fatty acid ratios and proportions.

Table 3; Percentage of fatty acids, their ratios (saturated and polyunsaturated fatty acids) and energy supply in calories (kcal/100g of food) contained in lipids of animal and vegetable origin.

SOURCES	Total AGS1(%)	Total PUFA2	PUFA/AGS ratio	n-6 Total	n-3 Total	Calories (Kcal/ 100g)
ANIMAL						
Beef tallow	47,4	3,7	0,08	3,1	0,6	902
Lard	38,9		0,29	10,2	1,0	902
swine		11,2				
Poultry fat	28,6	20,5	0,71	19,5	1,0	900
FISH OIL						
Salmon	18,6	47,4	2,55	2,1	31,4	902
VEGETABLE OILS						
Canola	5,8	29,6	5,10	20,3	9,3	884
Palma	48,9	9,3	0,19	9,1	0,2	884
Soy	14,2	57,8	4,07	51,0	6,8	884
Sunflower	8,9	40,0	4,49	39,8	0,2	884

1 SFA: saturated fatty acid; 2 PUFA: polyunsaturated fatty acid;

Source: Adapted from França, 2009

Certain vegetable oils (canola, flax, soy) contain a significant amount of ALA, the precursor of EPA and DHA. However, the latter are only found in concentrated form in fish oils (in different proportions depending on the fish) and algae (GRANDJEAN,

2006).

5.2.2-- Omega 6 fatty acids

The omega 6 fatty acids are biologically indispensable fatty acids and are all derived from an essential fatty acid, containing 18 carbon atoms and 2 double chemical bonds, called linoleic acid. Two other long-chain fatty acids, called gamma linolenic acid (GLA) and arachidonic acid, are derived from the latter. Indispensable for the synthesis of prostaglandins, molecules of hormonal activity, omega 6 fatty acids act on the health of the skin and the quality of the coat, as well as the animal's reproductive system. Vegetable oils are generally rich in omega-6 fatty acids. But some pork fats, and especially poultry fats, are also sources of large quantities of linoleic acid (more than 20% in poultry fat), as is egg yolk. On the other hand, bovine fats (lard, butter) contain very little of this nutrient (GRANDJEAN, 2006).

5.3 - Carbohydrates

Dogs, like other animals, have a metabolic need for glucose. Almost all commercial dog food contains starch, which, when hydrolyzed during digestion, will provide an ample supply of glucose. However, on a meat-based diet, with no carbohydrate intake, the dog meets its needs from gluconeogenesis in the liver and kidneys using precursors such as amino acids from proteins or glycerol from triglycerides to synthesize glucose. Therefore, carbohydrates do not seem to be essential in dog food, as long as there are enough gluconeogenic precursors, such as alanine, glycine or serine (POND, 2005).

The carbohydrates used in animal feed include high and low molecular weight sugars, starches, cell wall polysaccharides and dietary fibers. Functionally, the four groups of carbohydrates are: absorbable (monosaccharides such as glucose and fructose), digestible (disaccharides and oligosaccharides), fermentable (some oligosaccharides such as lactose) and non-fermentable (insoluble fibers such as cellulose) (KAHN, 2010).

Carbohydrates are a source of energy; one gram of carbohydrate generates approximately 3.5 kcal ME. Carbohydrate sources typically used in animal feed include rice, corn, potatoes, wheat, oats, barley, quinoa and sorghum. Vegetables are also considered a source of carbohydrates but have lower digestibility, common to starches with a high fiber content, such as most vegetables. The source and type of processing determines the digestibility of the carbohydrate. Rice is highly digestible for dogs, but wheat, oats and potatoes are poorly digested. Corn has a worse digestibility compared to rice. Cooking therefore increases the digestibility of all starches (SHENCK, 2010).

Different carbohydrate sources have different physiological effects. Properly cooked, non-fibrous carbohydrates are well utilized by dogs. However, if they are not cooked properly, they are poorly digested by dogs, which can cause flatulence and diarrhea (KAHN, 2010).

Sugars are sometimes added to feed and can be highly digestible in small quantities. Sucrose, found in molasses, honey, refined sugar, fruit and vegetables, is hydrolyzed in the small intestine to glucose and fructose. Lactose, found in milk and dairy products, is digested by the enzyme lactase. Lactase activity decreases when there is little lactose intake at weaning (SHENCK, 2010).

Carbohydrates are stored in the body to a limited extent as glycogen. If they are consumed in excess, they are stored as fat through the process of lipogenesis. Even if dogs don't have a minimum requirement for carbohydrates, they are used as "protein savers". As long as there is an adequate energy supply, provided by carbohydrates and/or fats, proteins can be used for tissue repair and growth (SHENCK, 2010).

Dogs normally tolerate high levels of carbohydrates without any problems. However, if excessive in their diet, carbohydrates can cause diarrhea because the intestine cannot digest and absorb all the sugar available. Some dogs may also have insufficient enzymatic activity when digesting carbohydrates (SHENCK, 2010).

Some studies carried out by different researchers on the use and utilization of starch in pets have shown that, in most extruded feeds for dogs and cats, starches are the main source of energy. They can represent between 40% and 55% of the dry matter in these feeds, providing between 30% and 60% of their metabolizable energy. Their nutritional characteristics depend on the composition of their sugars, their types of chemical bond, physico-chemical digestion factors and their processing (CARCIOFI, 2008).

Fiber is the name given to the sum of all plant polysaccharides in the diet (cellulose, hemicellulose, pectins, gums and mucilages), plus lignin, which are not hydrolyzed by the enzymes in the digestive tract of higher animals. The concept of fiber, originally defined as indigestible plant remains, has evolved over the last two decades. Nutritionists now classify fibres into water-soluble and non-water-soluble fractions and recognize the importance of fibre fermentation in the colon. Recently, the concept of fiber has been expanded to include fiber-like substances such as inulin, fructooligosaccharides and resistant starch. Thus, fibers contain many compounds with diverse physical and chemical properties (HUSSEIN, 2003, NESTLÉ, 2003a and 2003b).

Fiber types vary widely in their water-solubility, viscosity, ability to retain water and to bind minerals and organic molecules. These different characteristics result in various physiological effects (BORGES ET AL).

Insoluble fibers (lignin, cellulose and hemicellulose) are very poorly fermented by the intestinal flora and are excreted largely intact. By retaining water, they increase fecal mass and stool weight. These fibers have the effect of giving consistency to the fecal bolus, stimulating intestinal peristalsis. Because of their consistency, they tend to reduce intestinal transit time (NESTLÉ, 2003b).

Soluble fibers (pectins, gums, mucilages, beta-glucan and hemicellulose) act as substrates for fermentation in the colon, altering the microflora and physiology of the colon. In the proximal gastrointestinal tract, they have an effect on gastric emptying and absorption in the small intestine. They are also thickening agents and this property tends to increase the viscosity of the food bolus, decreasing the rate of gastric emptying and causing satiety and impact on food intake. Thus, in the proximal gastrointestinal tract, soluble fiber modifies satiety, modifies carbohydrate metabolism (reducing the glycemic response), and modifies lipid metabolism. In the colon, they are fermented and alter the composition of the intestinal flora and metabolism through the production of short-chain fatty acids (SCFA) or volatile fatty acids (VFA) (NESTLÉ, 2003b).

As this type of fiber can reduce postprandial levels of glucose, triglycerides and cholesterol in the blood, they are especially important in therapeutic diets, such as for obese or diabetic dogs (HUSSEIN, 2003).

Acetate, propionate and butyrate are the main VFA produced by fiber fermentation. The first consequence of this VFA production is the acidification of the colon, which can prevent the excessive proliferation of unwanted bacteria (e.g. clostridia). Acetate and most of the propionate reach the liver via the portal blood. Butyrate is absorbed by colon cells and used as "readily available energy" by these cells. The absorption of butyrate is coupled with the reabsorption of sodium and water, and may thus provide an anti-diarrheal effect. This is supported by evidence obtained in malnourished rats, in which the absence of butyrate production induced "starvation diarrhea" because the reabsorption of water and sodium was decreased. The feeding of enterocytes and colonocytes by VFA leads to hypertrophy of the intestinal mucosa, an increase in its weight and surface area, which optimizes the digestibility of nutrients by expanding their absorption surface. Animals receiving moderately fermentable fiber showed an increase in colon size, greater mucosal surface area and mucosal hypertrophy when compared to animals receiving non-fermentable fiber. The effect of VFA on colonic cell integrity and water reabsorption may be of crucial importance in antibiotic-associated diarrhea, when the normal flora is affected by the drug. Soluble fibers can help control excessive bacterial proliferation by maintaining VFA levels that acidify colon contents, providing energy to colon cells, maintaining intestinal integrity and supporting the development of normal healthy bacteria at the expense of pathogenic bacteria.

Some soluble fibers (such as inulin and other fructooligosaccharides) are preferentially fermented by bifidobacteria and lactobacilli and increase the level of these healthy bacteria in the microflora. This has been called the "prebiotic effect" (BORGES ET AL).

Dietary fiber (especially highly fermentable soluble fiber) promotes the development of colonic epithelium in rats, as shown by an increase in the mucosal DNA (Deoxyribonucleic Acid), RNA (Ribonucleic Acid) and protein content. For dogs and cats, the NRC (1985) and NRC (1986) do not recommend the minimum levels of fiber indicated or their limitations. Most commercial feeds have a fiber content of between 1 % and 4 % of dry matter, with the exception of therapeutic products. According to Hussein (2003), high levels of fiber (5 to 25% of DM) can be included in diets for obese dogs and in diets for healthy animals weighing within the standard range, when they are fed at will.

According to Sunvold et al. (1995), highly fermentable fiber can cause digestive disorders (high gas production), and a sudden change in the fiber source can cause a temporary imbalance, with uncontrolled fermentation, flatus and diarrhea. The high fermentability of some fibers can increase the volume of VFA, with an increase in their osmotic concentration and leakage of liquid into the intestinal lumen, causing gas and diarrhea.

Insoluble fibers, on the other hand, have an "aggressive" action on the muscles of the intestinal wall, which react by increasing their contractions (peristalsis), causing an increase in the speed of passage of the digestive tract and a decrease in the absorption of nutrients with a greater fecal residue or even diarrhea. In addition, these fibers can cause cryptitis, inflammation of the microvilli in the colon (PREMIERPET, 2003a).

Table 4 - Fermentation of dietary fiber for dogs.

FIBER TYPE	SOLUBILITY	FERMENTABILITY
Beet pulp	Low	Moderate
Citrus pulp	Low	Moderate
Cellulose	Low	Low
Rice bran	Low	Moderate
Aràbica gum	High	Moderate
Pectin	Low	High
Cabbage	Low	High

Adapted from Borges and Nunes (1998).

6 - Micronutrients

These are nutrients that are present in the diet in small quantities, but are of fundamental importance for the correct functioning of the animal organism. These are vitamins and minerals (EDNEY, 1989).

6.1 - Vitamins

Vitamins are important components of animal feed and are required for the normal functioning of all the body's systems. Vitamins are divided into two families: fat-soluble vitamins, which include vitamins A, D, E and K, which are stored in body fat, and water-soluble vitamins, which include the B-complex and C vitamins. If consumed in excess, fat-soluble vitamins can accumulate in the body and become toxic, while water-soluble vitamins are eliminated in the urine. Vitamins are supplied by different ingredients in food and can also be included in purified form. Each vitamin is involved in several different functions. Some vitamins are easily destroyed by cooking, so vitamin supplements should be added to the "feed" after the other ingredients have been cooked (SCHENCK, 2010).

6.1.1- Vitamin A (RETINOL)

Vitamin A is a fat-soluble vitamin that is important for vision and skin maintenance. Signs of deficiency can include: decreased night vision, opacity of the cornea, dehydration and skin lesions and atrophy of the sebaceous glands. Signs of poisoning are remodeling, lameness and death. Fish liver oil contains high levels of vitamin A; milk, liver and egg yolk are also rich sources of this vitamin; dogs can convert carotenoids (SCHENCK, 2010 & GRANDJEAN, 2006).

6.1.2- Vitamin D (CALCIFEROL)

It is fat-soluble and necessary for normal bone growth. Signs of deficiency include bone malformation, rickets (rare in dogs) and osteomalacia (muscle/joint pain and bone cracks). Signs of intoxication include dental abnormalities and bone deposition in soft tissues such as muscles and cartilage. In large breed puppies, excess vitamin D is much more common than deficiency, due to the indiscriminate use of supplements. There are few foods that are rich sources of vitamin D, meat and vegetables are practically devoid. Natural sources are cod liver oil, oily fish (tuna and sardines), egg yolk, milk and its derivatives. Dogs and cats do not synthesize vitamin D through exposure to sunlight on the skin, so their diet must be "supplemented" in order to adequately meet their requirements. Vitamin D deficiency results in secondary (nutritional) hyperparathyroidism, the most common problem resulting from poorly formulated homemade diets. (SCHENCK, 2010)

6.1.3- Vitamin E

Vitamin E is a fat-soluble vitamin that acts as a biological antioxidant and is required for normal reproduction. Vitamin E deficiency can lead to decreased reproductive performance, retinal degeneration and damage to the immune system. There are no reports of vitamin E-related toxicity. Rich sources of this vitamin include wheat germ, corn oil, soybean oil and sunflower oil. Egg yolk can also provide some amount of vitamin E. (SCHENCK, 2010)

6.1.4- Vitamin K

Vitamin K is a fat-soluble vitamin necessary for blood clotting. It is not added to feed because the bacteria in the intestine are able to synthesize all the vitamin K needed. Bleeding is the main sign of vitamin K deficiency. There is no known vitamin K toxicity. Foods with high levels of vitamin K include leafy green vegetables such as spinach, cabbage, kale and cauliflower, as well as liver and eggs. The bacteria in the large intestine can synthesize vitamin K, but prolonged treatment with antimicrobials can cause changes in the intestinal flora (Schenck, 2010).

6.1.5. - Vitamin B1 (Thiamine)

Thiamine is very important for the functioning of the nervous system. Its deficiency is caused by the ingestion of thiaminases, typical in diets containing raw fish. Signs of deficiency include incoordination, weakness and convulsions. There is no known toxicity. Some foods rich in thiamine are pork, beef, liver, wheat germ and some vegetables (SCHENCK, 2010).

6.1.6- Vitamin B2 (RIBOFLAVINE)

Riboflavin is important in many enzymatic reactions of metabolism. Signs of deficiency include decreased reproductive performance, dry skin, weakness and anemia. There is no known toxicity. Foods rich in riboflavin include milk, kidneys, liver, whole grains and vegetables (SCHENCK, 2010).

6.1.7- Vitamin B6 (PYRIDOXINE)

Pyridoxine is important in the formation of blood components and other metabolic proteins. Signs of deficiency are anemia and convulsions. There is no known toxicity. Foods rich in pyridoxine include liver, kidneys, fish, wheat germ and whole grains (SCHENCK, 2010).

6.1.8- Vitamin B12 (COLABAMINE)

It is important for blood formation and myelin synthesis. Deficiency is unlikely, except for rare genetic inheritance. Malabsorption disorders can be observed in Giant Schnauzers, Border Collies and Beagles. No toxicity is known. Vitamin B12 is only found in animal products, including red meat, poultry, fish and dairy products (SCHENCK, 2010).

6.1.9- Vitamin C

Vitamin C is required in the diet of pigs, primates (including humans) and other species. However, it is not included in the diet of dogs because they are able to synthesize it in the liver. Vitamin C is important in the synthesis of collagen and various other metabolic reactions, including the proper functioning of the immune system. Signs of deficiency include impaired healing, increased susceptibility to infections and muscle and joint pain. There is no known toxicity (SCHENCK, 2010).

6.2 - Minerals

Minerals are classified as macro and microminerals. Microminerals are present in small quantities (mg/kgh or ppm), but are indispensable for the functioning of the animal organism and include iron, zinc, copper, manganese, iodine and selenium. The macrominerals are present in higher quantities, namely calcium, phosphorus, magnesium, potassium, sodium and chlorine. Interactions occur between these minerals, so an excess of one mineral can result in a deficiency of another. Feed must be well formulated and developed to maintain an adequate balance between minerals.

6.2.1- Calcium (Ca)

Calcium is important for the formation and maintenance of bones and teeth. Signs of deficiency include lameness, bone demineralization and an increased incidence of fractures. During lactation, signs include convulsions and tetany (eclampsia). Excessive calcium intake results in growth retardation and severe bone and joint abnormalities. The ratio of calcium (Ca) to phosphorus (P) is very important for skeletal development. In recent years, there has been an increase in cases of ossification disorders in puppies of large dogs that consume industrialized food of inferior quality, due to the excess of minerals contained in this category of food. Foods rich in calcium include mammal bones, dairy products and vegetables. Grains, meat and offal have low levels of calcium, although it can still be found in mineral sources such as calcium carbonate or calcium phosphate (SCHENCK, 2010 & GRANDJEAN, 2006).

6.2.2- Phosphorus (P)

Phosphorus is also important in the formation and maintenance of bones and teeth. Eighty-six percent of the body's phosphorus is incorporated into the skeleton, to which it gives its solidity, in association with calcium. It is also a component of cell membranes and an element without which the body cannot use energy (through ATP). Phosphorus is also incorporated into large molecules such as DNA and

RNA, which carries the genetic material of cells. Deficiency of this mineral is rare, the characteristic sign being a poor appetite. Excess phosphorus generally occurs in animals fed strictly carnivorous diets, resulting in calcium deficiency and possible kidney damage. Foods rich in phosphorus include fish, red meat, poultry and wolves, as well as mammal bones and mineral salts such as phosphates. To limit the amount of phosphorus in the diet, part of the animal protein can be replaced by vegetable protein (soy protein, for example) (SCHENCK, 2010 & GRANDJEAN, 2006).

6.2.3- Potassium (K)

Potassium is important for maintaining water balance, some enzymatic reactions, nerve impulses and heart function. Lack of potassium results in loss of appetite, weakness, apathy, incoordination and paralysis. Toxicity does not usually occur, except when there is kidney failure and potassium is not excreted. Excess potassium is toxic to the heart and can lead to death. Meat, poultry, fish and some vegetables are rich in potassium (SCHENCK, 2010).

6.2.4- Sodium (Na)

Sodium is important for maintaining water balance, nerve cells and muscle fibers. Signs of deficiency are poor appetite, weight loss and stunted growth. High levels of sodium in the diet result in increased urinary excretion and water consumption. However, signs of intoxication include convulsions and death. However, sodium intake does not pose a particular problem, as dogs do not sweat even during intense physical exertion. Dairy products, red meat, poultry, fish and eggs are foods rich in sodium (SCHENCK, 2010).

6.2.5- Chlorine (Cl)

Chlorine is important for maintaining hydroelectrolyte balance and acid-base balance. Chlorine deficiency or excess usually occurs in pathological states, episodes of prolonged vomiting, kidney disease, etc. Foods rich in sodium are the same as those rich in chlorine (SCHENCK, 2010).

6.2.6- Magnesium (Mg)

Magnesium is important for the normal function of muscles and nerves. Signs of deficiency include weakness, convulsions and death. Excess magnesium can cause diarrhea. Whole grains, legumes and dairy products are rich in magnesium, as are the bones of mammals (SCHENCK, 2010 & GRANDJEAN, 2006).

6.2.7- Sulphur (S)

Sulphur is necessary for the synthesis of chondroitin sulphate (found in cartilage), insulin, heparin and glutathione (immunomodulator and antioxidant). It is a constituent of biotin and thiamine (vitamins), and amino acids such as cisterna and methionine. The sulphur present in the diet is poorly absorbed, but there is no deficiency due to adequate consumption of cysteine and methionine (SCHENCK, 2010).

6.2.8- Iron (Fe)

Iron is important in the formation of blood cells. It is the indispensable component of hemoglobin, the pigment that ensures oxygen transport in red blood cells (RBCs) and myoglobin (muscles). Iron deficiency results in anemia. Signs of toxicity include weight loss, loss of appetite and death. Iron-rich foods include liver, kidneys, egg yolk, fish, green vegetables and whole grains (SCHENCK, 2006; GRANDJEAN, 2010).

6.2.9- Copper (Cu)

Copper is necessary for the transport of iron and the formation of red blood cells. Copper deficiency also results in anemia. Excess copper can cause kidney damage. The foods richest in copper are meats (lamb, pork and duck) and legumes (lentils, peas and soybeans) (SCHENCK, 2006; GRANDJEAN, 2010).

6.2.10 - Manganese (Mn)

Manganese is important for reproductive function and joint formation. Deficiency signs include a drop in reproductive performance, abortion, stiffness and bone abnormalities. An excess of this mineral also results in a decline in reproductive function. Legumes and whole grains are rich in manganese (SCHENCK, 2010).

6.2.11 - Zinc (Zn)

Zinc is important for the formation and maintenance of the skin, sense of taste and immune function. Deficiency leads to scabs and skin lesions, dryness and dullness of the hair, retarded growth, a drop in reproductive function, atrophy of the testicles and diarrhea. Excess zinc causes vomiting and can lead to calcium and copper deficiency. Zinc is found in whole grains and all animal products. If supplementation is necessary, zinc can be supplied in organic form (zinc gluconate or zinc-methionine) to facilitate absorption (SCHENCK, 2010; GRANDJEAN, 2006).

6.2.12 - Iodine (I)

Iodine is important for maintaining thyroid function. Iodine deficiency causes thyroid disorders, hair loss and drowsiness. Excess iodine also causes thyroid disorders (SCHENCK, 2010).

6.2.13 - Selenium (Se)

Selenium is important for maintaining muscle function. Signs of deficiency include skeletal disorders, weakness and heart disease. An excess of selenium can result in vomiting, weakness and death. Grains, meat and fish are foods rich in this mineral (SCHENCK, 2010).

6.2.14 - Chromium (Cr)

Chromium is an insulin catalyst. Chromium deficiency is associated with the development of diabetes (SCHENCK, 2010).

7 - INGREDIENTS USED IN DOG FOOD.

7.1 - Meat

When it comes to meat, it is considered to be made up of muscle tissue, accompanied by intramuscular and subcutaneous fat, connective tissue, tendons and blood vessels. The relative proportion between muscle fibers and connective tissue has a great influence on the texture and tenderness of the meat, however, the real differences in nutrient content between meats are more related to the amount of fat. Lean meat has a constant proportion of water and protein, 75% water and 25% protein, regardless of whether it is from different parts of the same animal or from different animals such as cattle, sheep, pigs or poultry. Raw lean meat from cows, chickens, sheep, pigs, ducks and rabbits has a very similar composition, with averages for water, protein and fat ranging from 70-76%, 20-22% and 2-9% respectively. Fat varies the most, with poultry, beef and pork having less fat (2-5%) than sheep meat (79%) (EDNEY, 1989).

Since the proportions of fat vary widely between the different parts of the same carcass, and between different animals, it is impossible to make exact estimates of the protein, fat and energy content of a given piece of meat from food composition tables. The quality of the protein in the meat of all mammals and birds is of high biological value. Therefore, it is difficult to choose one in terms of nutrient content among the meats of different animals (EDNEY, 1989).

Meat by-products such as the liver, kidneys and spleen often have the same amount of nutrients, regardless of the species. However, there are big differences in nutrient content between them, for example, the liver has a different content to the spleen. They usually have varying levels of fat and vitamins, depending on the food consumed by the animals. All meats have a low calcium content, with very different calcium:phosphorus ratios, ranging from 1:15 to 1:26. All muscle meats and some veal (by-products) are deficient in iodine and vitamins A and D. The liver and kidney, to a lesser extent, are sources of these vitamins. In fact, the liver contains so much vitamin A (retinol) that cats show hypervitaminosis when fed liver-based diets (EDNEY, 1989).

Meat is a good source of good quality protein and fat, iron and some B vitamins, especially niacin, thiamine, riboflavin and vitamin B12. They are highly palatable and acceptable to dogs, and often have high digestibility, which means that the nutrients are easily utilized by the body. If properly supplemented with calcium, phosphorus, iodine and vitamins A and D, they are excellent food (EDNEY, 1989).

Meat by-products include materials such as blood, meaty bones, heads and extremities of butchered animals. Bearing in mind that these products can include bone and have a high calcium and phosphorus content, they can be used to correct deficiencies in products such as muscle meat or other by-products like liver and lungs. These products are not very suitable for use in homemade diets, as they are used raw, increasing the risk of biological contamination, although they are widely used in the manufacture of commercial feed (EDNEY, 1989).

7.2 - Dairy Products

Cream, skimmed milk, whey, yogurt, cheese and butter are dairy products that contain more of the nutrients of the original milk. They are generally well accepted by dogs. Some individuals cannot tolerate more than a minimal amount of milk sugar (lactose), and because they have insufficient amounts of the enzyme (lactase), they may suffer from diarrhea (EDNEY, 1989).

Milk contains most of the nutrients needed in a dog's diet. However, there is little iron and vitamin D. The riboflavin present in milk is sensitive to sunlight and most of it is destroyed, as is vitamin C (not essential for dogs), if exposed for more than an hour or two. Milk is a good source of energy, easily utilized, high quality protein, fat, carbohydrates, calcium, phosphorus and various other trace elements, vitamin A, D, E and B vitamins (EDNEY, 1989).

7.3 - Eggs

Eggs are a good source of iron, protein, riboflavin, folic acid, vitamin B12 and vitamins A and D. They also contain considerable amounts of most nutrients, except vitamin C and carbohydrates. Contrary to popular belief, the differences between the nutritional values of eggs, due to the production system, are very small. They may affect the content of folic acid and vitamin B12, but very little of the rest of the components. Eggs are usually eaten without shells, even though shells are a good source of calcium, since they consist of calcium carbonate and proteins. Despite this, shelled eggs are excellent food. Egg whites consist almost exclusively of protein and water, with trace elements and some B vitamins. Most of the B vitamins and all the fat-soluble ones are found in the yolk, which contains more fat and protein and much less water than the white. Eggs contain very little niacin (EDNEY, 1989).

The white of raw eggs contains avidin, a substance that prevents the action and absorption of biotin. It is therefore not recommended to feed raw eggs frequently to dogs. Cooking destroys the inhibitory effect of biotin. Cooked egg whites are more digestible and there are no advantages to giving raw eggs. In addition, raw eggs may be related to cases of diarrhea in dogs (EDNEY, 1989).

7.4 - Other animal products

There are many by-products from the slaughterhouse that can be used as food for dogs and cats. Some are obtained fresh, others are part of previously processed animals. These include dehydrated meals such as blood meal, meat meal, meat and bone meal and bone meal. All these products enter the animal feed trade and are also produced with certain protein, fat and ash contents. The quality of the protein and its uses can be variable, as can the content of ash or mineral matter. They provide large amounts of protein, ranging from 40% in some meat and bone meals to 75-80% in quality meat meals. Digestibility for dogs can be as high as 90% and as low as 70%. They are generally very well accepted and improve the acceptability of cereals when mixed. Their main use is as part of industrialized dry foods. Sterilized bone meal can be used in natural or homemade feed. Bone meal contains approximately 32% calcium and 14% phosphorus, making it a good calcium and phosphorus supplement for meat; 15 grams is enough to supplement 1 kilogram of meat (EDNEY, 1989).

7.5 - Cherries

Cereals are the seeds of grains. They include wheat, barley, oats, rice, rye, corn and sorghum. Cereal grains are made up of the germ and the embryo, surrounded by a starchy endosperm, whose function is to provide carbohydrates (starch) and proteins (germ) for the embryo. The endosperm is surrounded by a layer of aleurone, which is a thin layer of cells rich in protein and phosphorus, on top of which is the outermost layer of the seed. During the milling process, the different layers are separated so that the bran is the outermost layer and includes polysaccharides, cellulose and hemicellulose, the flour is the endosperm and the germ is the embryo (EDNEY, 1989).

Whole grains of the most common cereals, such as wheat, oats, barley, rice and wheat, contain approximately 12% moisture, 9-14% protein, 2-5% fat and 70-80% carbohydrates in the form of starch. Wheat, oats and barley have a higher protein content and lower fat content than corn and rice. In general, their value as food for dogs and cats is as a source of energy (EDNEY, 1989).

Rice found in the supermarket is made up of whole grains from which the outer layer has been removed and is made up of approximately 85% starch, with small amounts of vitamins, minerals, fat and protein. Rice must be properly cooked and mixed with other more palatable ingredients before being offered to animals (EDNEY, 1989).

7.6 - Vegetable Products

Plant products can be classified into three groups, taking into account their use as food. Firstly, those in which the whole plant, stalks and leaves are used. These include lettuce, cabbage, Brussels sprouts and cauliflower, etc., which can be eaten raw or cooked. They have a high water content, a high fiber content and, although they are important in human diets, they are of little value to dogs. They are not very acceptable for dogs and their volume and poorly digestible fiber content mean that large quantities would have to be consumed for them to constitute a significant part of the nutrient intake. Dogs can obtain certain amounts of vitamin A from these vegetables. They are also rich in B vitamins, but they can be destroyed by cooking or lost in the liquid used in the process if it is not given to the animals (EDNEY, 1989).

The second group is made up of roots and tubers. These are the storage organs of plants, made up of starch. Some examples are potatoes, carrots and turnips. Roots eaten raw are poorly digested by dogs and are usually not offered. Cooking gelanitizes the starch and makes it more digestible, so most dogs consume cooked potatoes and carrots. Their nutritional value is as a source of energy, although carrots can provide dogs with certain amounts of vitamin A. There are no risks in giving these vegetable products to dogs (EDNEY, 1989).

The third group is made up of those vegetables from which the seeds are consumed. These include beans and peas. They are relatively rich in protein and provide more energy than green and root vegetables, with the exception of potatoes. They are a good source of B vitamins. Peas and beans are well accepted by dogs if they are cooked, however, they are rarely included as an important part of the diet. Soybeans are a special case. They are an important source of protein and energy for humans in many parts of the world, and are currently used in animal feed, after the olive oil process. The seeds have an outer layer, or husk, which is removed by mechanical methods before the oil extraction process begins, carried out by grinding and treatment with solvents. The extraction residue contains the protein, carbohydrate and mineral portions, with a small amount of oil. In order to inactivate certain anti-nutritional factors (anti-trypsins and hemagglutinins), the seeds are heat-treated, i.e. roasted. Defatted and toasted soy flour has a protein content of 48-50%,   30% carbohydrates in the form of non-starch sugars, 1-2% fat, approximately 5-6% minerals and 3-5% crude fiber. The protein is of high quality and contains high levels of essential amino acids (EDNEY, 1989).

Soy flour can be used directly as a raw material for some diets and can be processed to obtain soy protein. Most legumes contain complex carbohydrates and simpler sugars that are resistant to digestion by the enzymes of dogs, cats and humans. They reach the large intestine undigested and can undergo bacterial fermentation, with the consequent production of flatus and intestinal gas. The extent of fermentation and gas production resulting from the ingestion of soy, beans or peas depends on the quantities consumed and the susceptibility of the individual, which depends on the bacterial flora present in the intestine (EDNEY, 1989).

8 - RECIPE FOR AN ADULT DOG

A recipe was formulated using software (BalanceIT ®), simulating the needs of a 3-year-old adult male, neutered canine, weighing 25 kilograms, with a body score of index 4, in a healthy state of maintenance. The software allows you to choose the ingredients to be used and calculates the possibilities of recipes that meet minimum needs, based on all the information mentioned. Below is a profile of the ingredients that make up the diet.

Table 5 . Dietary ingredient profile for an adult dog

INGREDIENTS	QUANTITY (gr)
Carrot	66,5
Italian zucchini	90
Pumpkin and its varieties	78,8
White rice	286,4
Minced beef, (second class)	262,2
Canola oil	3,9

Source: Adapted from Delaney (2004)

The recipe described above produces a meal with 1109 kcal, 30% protein (331 kcal), 37% fat (410 kcal), 33% carbohydrates (368 kcal) and 69.9% moisture. This is 101% of a dog's daily energy needs (DELANEY, 2004).

Instructions and method of preparation

According to Delaney et al. (2004), this recipe has exactly the amount of food to be offered each day, in more than one meal. The food can be prepared ahead of time and refrigerated for up to three days, or frozen for up to two weeks without losing its biological value. Minced meat should be cooked thoroughly without the addition of spices and condiments. Rice should be cooked without adding any seasoning. Vegetables, cut into small pieces, should be kept in hot water until they boil or should be steamed (ideal). Measure out the indicated amounts of minced meat, white rice and vegetables after they have been cooked, cutting up the vegetables. Put all the ingredients in a bowl and add the above amount of canola oil. The meal can be offered hot (more palatable) or cold, the supplements should be added before serving. Mix well and serve!

Ingredients should not be substituted without prior study, they can vary greatly in the amounts and types of nutrients they provide. This is especially true of vegetable oils, which have very specific fatty acid profiles and vitamin content. Canola oil, in particular, is rich in polyunsaturated fatty acids from the omega 3 and 6 series and in vitamin E.

The homemade diet is perfectly balanced, with the right proportion of ingredients. However, the software provides a complete list of the nutrients contained in the diet, and points out the deficiencies of this recipe for an adult dog in those conditions. The Ca:P ratio of the diet is 1:5.7, with deficiencies in some mineral salts, as well as some vitamins and essential amino acids, which are below nutritional requirements, requiring supplementation to supply the following amounts of nutrients:

- Calcium, 1.57 grams; Phosphorus, 0.65 grams; Potassium, 0.155 grams; Copper, 1.576 micrograms; Iodine, 0.38 micrograms; Iron, 12.208 micrograms; and Zinc, 16.408 micrograms;

- Vitamin D, 126,440 IU; Riboflavin (Vitamin B2), 0.69 micrograms; Choline, 105.065 micrograms; and Tryptophan, 0.025 grams.

1.1 - Natural Supplementation

Some natural supplements can be used to make up for deficiencies in these nutrients. Supplementation can be done with 50 grams of cooked beef liver, which according to TACO (2011), has 2 mg of Zinc, 155 mg of Potassium, 3 mg of Calcium, 210 mg of Phosphorus, 2.9 mg of Iron, 6.3 mg of Copper and 1.35 mg of Riboflavin. It meets the needs of Potassium, Copper, Riboflavin and Tryptophan, as this herb has high levels of these essential amino acids.

You can also add 4.2 grams of bone meal to the homemade diet, which according to Avelar et al. (2006) contains 1.54 grams of available calcium, as well as 588 mg of phosphorus, 478 mg of zinc and 900 mg of iron, meeting the needs of these minerals.

According to the USDA (2011), one teaspoon of cod liver oil contains approximately 450 IU of Vitamin D. Therefore, half a teaspoon would be enough to cover the vitamin D deficiency.

9 - DANGEROUS FOODS FOR DOGS

Chocolate and Coffee

Chocolate, coffee and their derivatives contain substances called methylxanthines and their by-products (such as treombomine), which are found in cocoa (Theobroma cacao). When ingested by animals, methylxanthines can cause vomiting, diarrhea, dyspnea, polyuria, polydpisia, hyperactivity, cardiac arrhythmias, tremors, convulsions and even death. The darker the chocolate, the more dangerous it is (ASPCA, 2012). Cases of sudden death have been reported following the ingestion of 300 grams of chocolate in Dachshunds and Springer Spaniels, 12 hours after ingestion (WILLS & SIMPSON).

Alcohol

Alcoholic beverages and products containing alcohol can cause vomiting, diarrhea, motor incoordination, central nervous system depression, difficulty breathing, tremors, coma and even death (ASPCA, 2012).

Avocado

Avocado leaves, fruits and seeds contain Persin, which can cause vomiting and diarrhea in dogs. Birds and rodents are especially sensitive to avocado poisoning, and can develop congestion, breathing difficulties and fluid accumulation around the heart (ASPCA, 2012).

Macadamia nuts

Macadamia nuts are used in foods and sweets. However, they can cause problems for canine companions. They cause weakness, tremors and hyperthermia in dogs. The signs usually appear 12 hours after ingestion and can last up to 48 hours (ASPCA, 2012).

Onion, garlic and chives

These legumes and vegetables can cause gastrointestinal irritation and can lead to hemolytic anemia. However, cats are more susceptible, dogs are at greater risk if larger quantities are consumed. Although cats are more susceptible, dogs are also at risk if a large enough quantity is consumed. Toxicity is usually diagnosed through history, clinical signs and microscopic confirmation of Heinz corpuscles (ASPCA, 2012). According to Wills & Simpson (1994), the ingestion of raw onions, equivalent to 30 grams, for three days produced hemolytic anemia, hemoglobinuria and hemoglobionemia.

10 - CONCLUSION

Dogs have been with us for thousands of years and are now completely dependent on man for the survival of the species, who provides for their needs, ranging from shelter and safety to food. The dog, a carnivorous animal, has adapted to the human way of life and today lives confined to the space of domestic homes. In the last 80 years, humans have started using commercial, balanced dog food, which for reasons of practicality is widely used to feed dogs. However, these feeds contain synthetic chemicals used as dyes, flavorings and preservatives, some of which are not proven to be safe for animals. They also contain ingredients that are less suitable for feeding carnivores (or semi-carnivores), as dogs are classified.

Food is of the utmost importance for maintaining life, energy availability, tissue composition and many other factors that affect the body. This work has shown how it is possible to feed dogs in a more natural and safer way, i.e. with high quality ingredients that more closely resemble those ingested by animals in the wild, without the addition of dubious chemical substances that put the animals' health at risk. In addition, natural food improves the quality of the coat, gently reduces the smell of animals, reduces the quantity and improves the quality of feces, is more acceptable and allows adaptation to different physiological and pathological states of the animal.

However, it is essential that the feed to be offered is properly balanced in terms of ingredient content, in order to avoid nutritional imbalances, as well as the correct use of supplements to correct any deficiencies and avoid an excess of certain nutrients. It is also recommended to formulate more than one diet, i.e. varying the ingredients, in order to offer a balanced, highly digestible diet with different sources of nutrients.

REFERENCES

ASPCA; People Foods to Avoid Feeding Your Pets; American Society for the Prevention of Cruelty to Animals (ASPCA): Poison Control;2012; Available at :http://www.aspca.org/pet-care/poison-control/people-foods.aspx> Accessed on: July 19, 2012.

NATIONAL ASSOCIATION OF PET FOOD MANUFACTURERS. **Manual do programa integrado de qualidade pet**. 2. ed. Sao Pulo, 2008. 238p.

AVELAR, A.C., FERREIRA, W.M.; BRITO, W.;MENEZES, M.A.B.C.; Mineral composition of phosphates, limestone and bone meal used in Brazilian agriculture; Department of Animal Science: UFMG Veterinary School; 2006; Belo Horizonte, Brazil.

BORGES, F.M.O.; SALGARELLO, R.M.; GURIAN, T.M.; Recent advances in dog and cat nutrition. 32f. Federal University of Lavras, MG.

CARCIOFI, A. C. Protein and carbohydrate sources for dogs and cats. Revista Brasileira de Zootecnia, Viçosa, MG, v. 37, p. 28-41, 2008. Special supplement.

CARCIOFI, A. C.; BAZZOLI, R. S.; ZANNI, A.; KIHARA, L. R.L.; PRADA, F. Influence of water content and the digestibility of pet foods on the water balance of cats. **Brazilian Journal Veterinary Research Animal Science,** Sâo Paulo, v. 42, n. 6, p. 429-434, 2005.

CASE, L. P.; CAREY, D. P.; HIDREAKAWA, D. A. **Canine and feline nutrition:** manual for professionals. Madrid: Harcourt Brace, 1998. 424p.

DELANEY, S. et al.; Balance it: Free Recipe Generator Powered by Auto Balancer ®;2004 Available at <https://secure.balanceit.com/tools/recipes/recipegenerator/>; Accessed on: July 19, 2012.

EDNEY, A.T.B.. The Waltham Book of Nutrition for Cats and Dogs. Zaragoza, Spain. Editora Acribia, second edition. 1989

FLAIM, D.; Natural Dog Food No-Nos. 2012. Available at <http://www.dogchannel.com/dog-magazines/dogfancy/dog-channel- exclusive/dog-fancy-exclusive-0808/natural-dog-food-no-nos.aspx >Accessed July 19, 2012.

FRANÇA, J.; Conventional versus natural food for adult dogs. 2009. 93pf. Thesis (PhD in Zootechnics), Zootechnics Postgraduate Program, University of Lavras, Lavras, MG.2009.

GODFREY, S; RUISH, D.; Evolutionary nutrition for the dog; Distributed by Going to the dogs Inc:

<hhttp://www.reddogdeli.com/pdfs/EvolutionaryNutritionfortheDog.pdf> Accessed July 20, 2012)

GRANDJEAN, D.; Everything you need to know about the role of nutrients in the health of dogs and cats. Aniwa Publishing, first edition. 96pg. 2006.

GROOT, J.; SHREUDER, W. **Biological, naturally logical**. Amsterdam: AFB International. Available at: <www.afbinternational.com/images/upload/biological,%20naturally% 20logical.pdf>. Accessed on: April 20, 2009.

HENDRIKSAN, W. H.; SRITHARAN, K. Apparent ileal and fecal digestibility of dietary protein is different in dogs. **Journal of Nutrition,** Philadelphia, v. 132, p.1692S-1694S, June 2002.

KAHN, C.M.; LINE, S.; The Mercky Veterinary Manual. John Wile & Sons: Tenth edition.2945pg. 2010.

MEEKER, D. L. **Essential rendering:** all about the animal by-products industry. Arlington: Kirby Lithographic Company, 2006. 302p.

NATIONAL RESEARCH COUNCIL. **Nutrient requirements of dogs and cats.** Washington: National Academies, 2006. 398 p.

NESTLÉ Fibers in enteral nutrition. Available at: http://nutricaoclinica.nestle.com.br, Accessed on: 03/06/2003b

NESTLÉ Soluble and insoluble fibers. Available at: http://nutricaoclinica.nestle.com.br, Accessed on: 03/06/2003a

POND, W.G.; CHURCH, D.C.; POND, K.R.; SCHOKNECHT, P.A.: Basic Animal Nutrition and Feeding. Wiley International, first edition. 2005.

SCHENCK, P.A.; Home-Prepared Dogs and Cats Diets; Wiley-blackwell, second edition, 546pg. 2010.

SUNVOLD, G.D., FAHEY, G.C. JR., MERCHEN, N.R., et al. Dietary Fiber for cats: In vitro fermentation of selected Fiber sources by cat fecal inoculum and In vivo utilization of diets containing selected Fiber sources and their blends. Journal of Animal Science, v.73, p.2329-2339.,1995.

PREMIER PET. Moderately Fermentable Fibers in Dog and Cat Food. Newsletter, Available at http://www.premierpet.com.br, Accessed on 13/10/2002a

TACO. **Brazilian Table of Food Composition**. University State of Campinas, 2011. Available at:

<http://www.unicamp.br/nepa/taco/home.php?ativo=home>. Accessed on: July 20, 2012.

USDA; National Nutrient Database for Standard References; United States Department of Agriculture: Human Nutrition Information Service; 2011; Available at: <http://ndb.nal.usda.gov/ndb/foods/show/674> Accessed on: July 20, 2012.

WILLS, J.M.; SIMPSON, K.W. The WALTHAM Book of CLINICAL NUTRITION of the Dog & Cat. Pergamon Publishing House: first edition; 1994

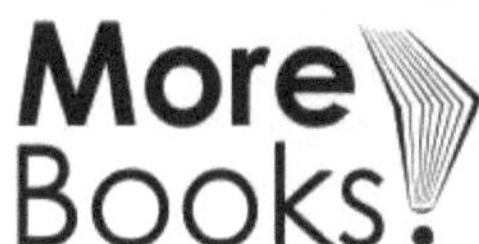

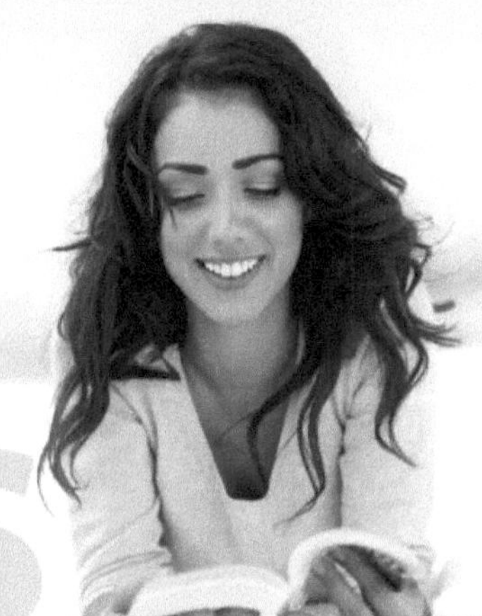

yes
I want morebooks!

Buy your books fast and straightforward online - at one of world's fastest growing online book stores! Environmentally sound due to Print-on-Demand technologies.

Buy your books online at
www.morebooks.shop

Kaufen Sie Ihre Bücher schnell und unkompliziert online – auf einer der am schnellsten wachsenden Buchhandelsplattformen weltweit! Dank Print-On-Demand umwelt- und ressourcenschonend produzi ert.

Bücher schneller online kaufen
www.morebooks.shop

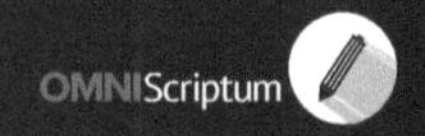

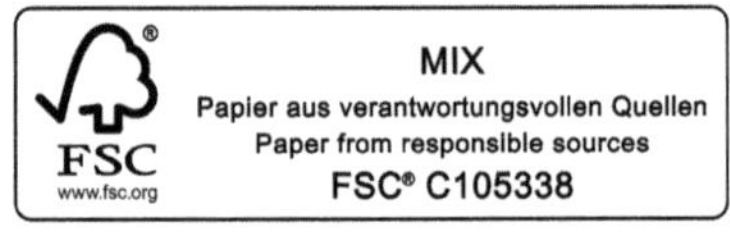

Printed by Books on Demand GmbH, Norderstedt / Germany